Life Blood
By Daniel A. DuBour

Life Blood is a complete description
Of where red blood cells are made
And their function
In the human
Body.

Simplificd
For all those unfamiliar with the
Purpose of the red blood cell
And how it works
In our bodies.

ISBN-13: 978-1505688979
ISBN-10: 1505688973

Life Blood
By Daniel A. DuBour

Contents

Life Blood
By Daniel A. DuBour

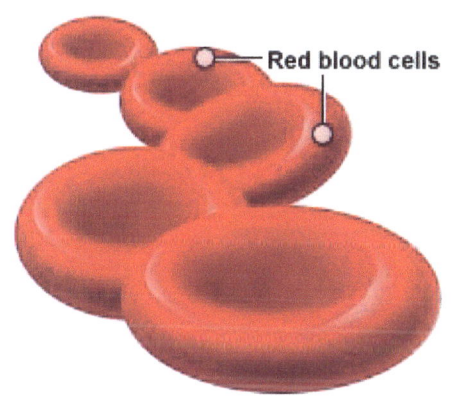

Red Blood Cells are shaped
Very much like a doughnut.
They are round and in the middle
Indented but no hole.

Where the cell is indented,
The Red Blood Cell
Can easily pick up and carry oxygen
And other nutrients;
Nourishment to the tissues
Throughout our body.

Blood cells are born in the center part of Our bones; it is called the bone morrow.

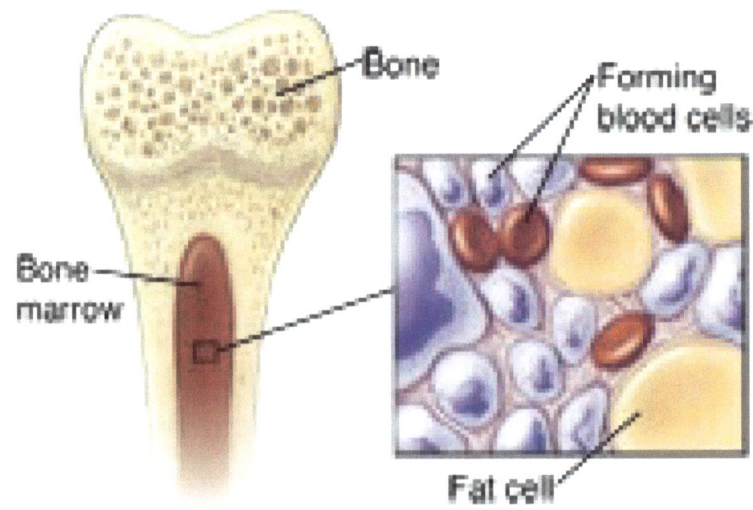

Once the blood cells are formed, they enter The blood stream; called the circulatory system.

Now the red blood cell goes to work.
But first it has to pick up the oxygen
From the lungs.
It's a good thing it has a pathway
To where it must go.

The pathway for blood to travel is called our
Veins and arteries.

Vein

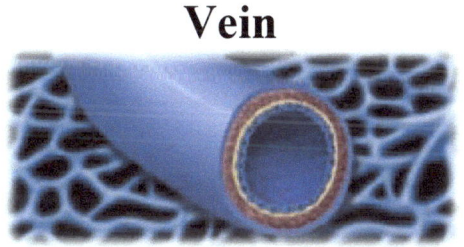

The vein is the pathway
Where the red blood cells
Carry waste material
From the body cells out of the body.

The red blood cells carry carbon dioxide
From the body cells to the lungs
Where the carbon dioxide goes
Into the air when we breathe out.

When we breathe in, our lungs take in oxygen.

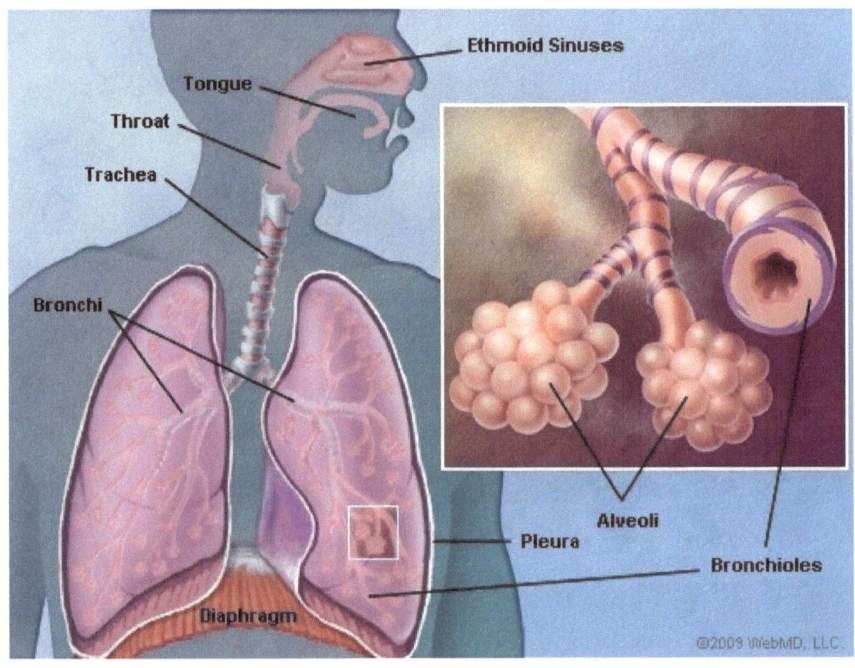

Once the red blood cell gets rid of the carbon dioxide
And is filled with the oxygen,
It goes back into circulation.

From the lungs,
Now filled with the nourishing Oxygen:

The red blood cells enter a pathway
Called Arteries.

Artery

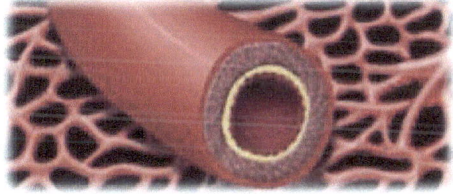

What makes these red blood cells to move in the
Veins and arteries?

Our Heart

Our Heart is the pump that forces
The
Red blood cells through our bodies
In pathways called Arteries.

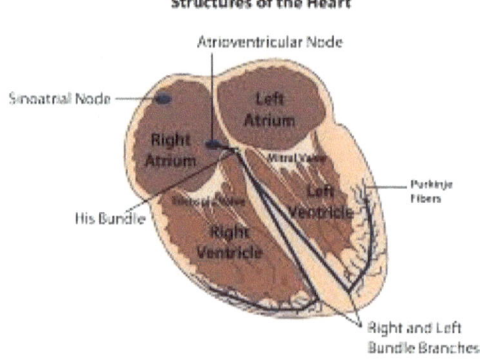

The heart is made up of four chambers.

There are two chambers in the heart named
Atriums.

They are located on the on the two top section
Of the heart.

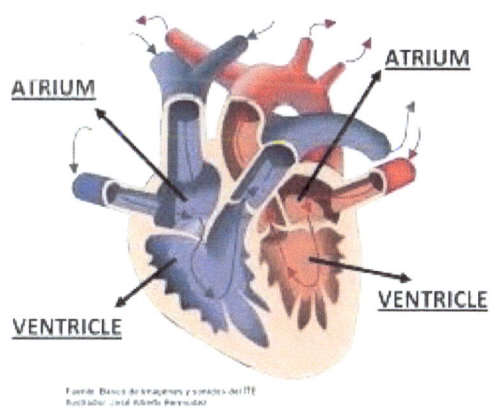

The atrium on the right side of the heart
Receives blood from the veins.

The atrium on the left side of the heart
Receives blood from the lungs
Filled with oxygen.

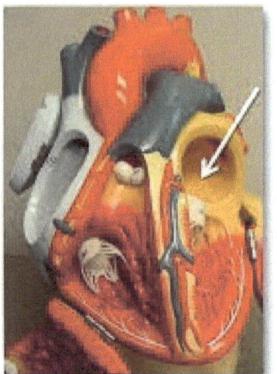

Left Atrium

**The blood is then forced through Valves
That Open and close.**

**The valve on the right side of the heart is
Called the tricuspid valve.**

**And the valve on the left side of the heart
Is called the mitral valve.**

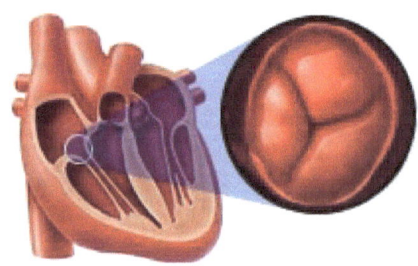

The tricuspid valve and the mitral valves
Open and close at the same time.

The blood forced through the valves of the atriums
Enters the two chambers of the heart called
Ventricles.

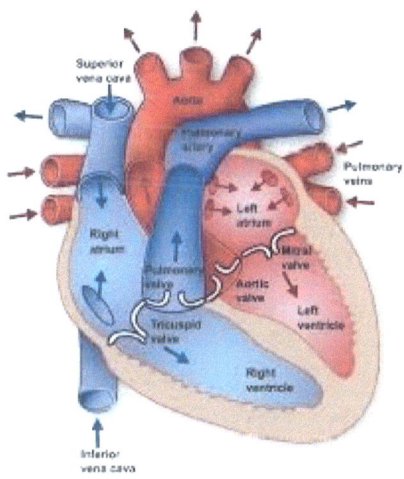

The blood in the right ventricle is forced to the
Lungs.

The blood in the left ventricle is forced throughout
The body.

You are probably wondering how this all work.
The heart is a very unique pump.
Actually;
It's a muscle with its own electrical
System.

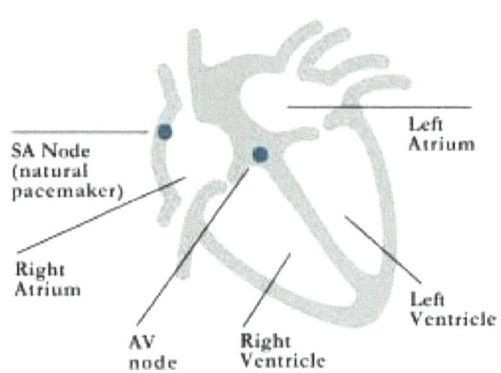

The SA Node on the right side of the heart
Delivers a shock which is sent to the AV node
This causes the ventricles to contract.
Forcing all the blood inside to move out.

When the ventricles contract,
The blood in both the
Right and the left ventricles
Are forced out of the chambers.

At the same time;
The atrium chambers are being filled
With blood.

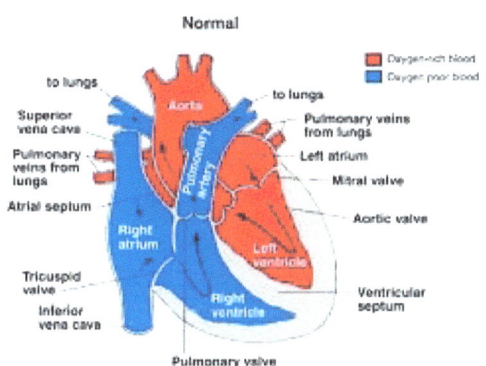

The blood cells on the right side of the heart
Is forced out of the ventricle
Into a vein pathway leading to the lungs
To release the carbon dioxide
And to receive Oxygen.

When we breathe out
The carbon dioxide is released into the air.

Oxygen is attached to the
Red blood cell
When we breathe in.

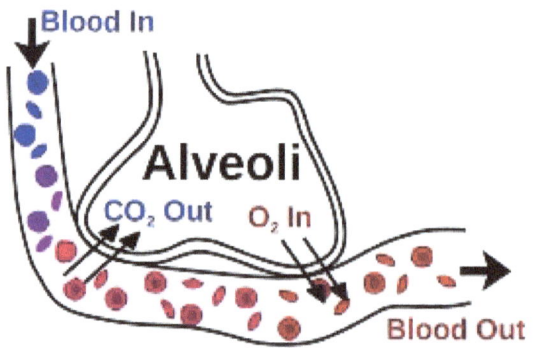

The red blood cells then travel to
Right Atrium of the heart.
When the heart is at "rest"

The blood cells in the right ventricles;
Now filled with
Oxygen from the lungs is forced into a large pathway
Called the Aorta.

The Aorta is the pathway to the arteries
Where the red blood
Cells flow throughout the body
To deliver oxygen
And nutrients to the body cells.

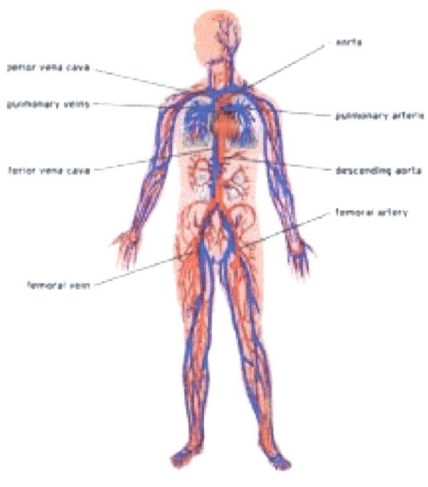

Once the red blood cells reach the cell tissues;
They enter tiny blood vessels called Capillaries.

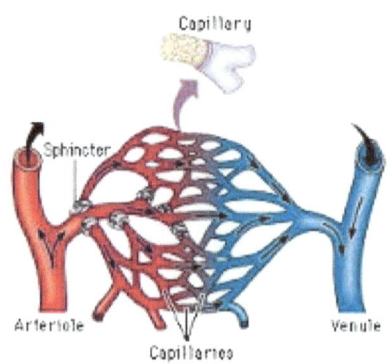

At this point the oxygen is delivered to the cell,
And the Cell in return gives off carbon dioxide
To the blood cell.

The blood cell then takes the waste material
For disposal
Through the pathway
Called veins.

The veins are the pathway
Where the red blood cells
Pass through to go back to the heart.

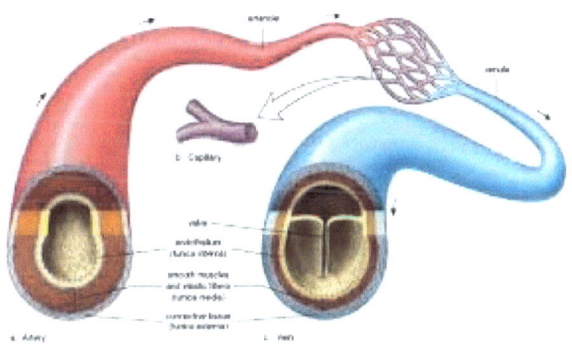

The red blood cell,
After completing its mission
Of delivering oxygen to the body cells
Returns to the heart and
Starts all over again.

Fun Facts

**There are 5,000,000 Red Blood Cells
In one drop of blood.
A young person has 1 gallon of blood,
And an adult has 5 quarts of blood
In their bodies.**

One Gallon

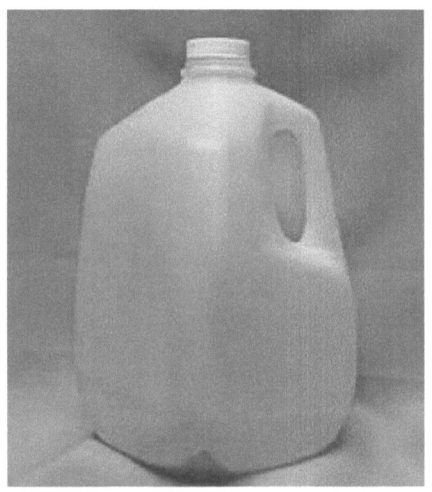

Five Quarts

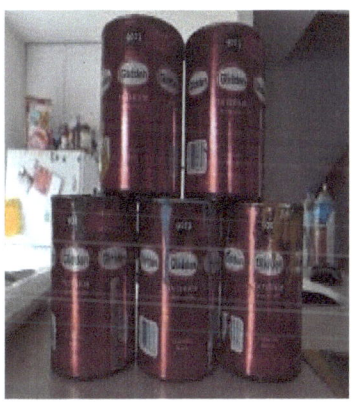

Red Blood Cells consist of liquids,
Solids and a small amount of Oxygen
And Carbon Dioxide.

Red Blood Cells flow in 90% water,
Nutrients and Proteins.

Now that you know
All about the Red Blood Cells
And how they are used in our bodies;
Now you should know
How to take care of your
Body to insure the Red Blood Cells
Can do the job affectively.

Nutrition:
Your body requires food for nourishment;
Meats,
Fish, cheese, bread products,
Water and vitamins.

Exercise regularly,
Walking and swimming are great!

Don't Smoke!

If you take care of your body,
You will have a long healthy life.

Food Groups

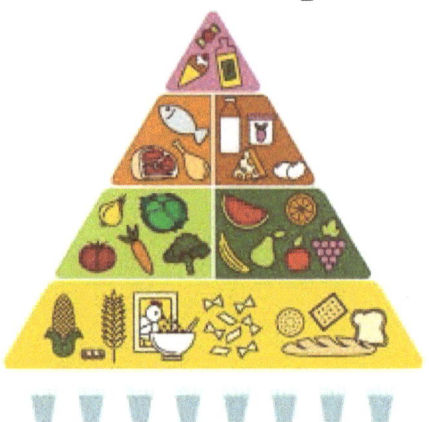

Start from the bottom of the triangle and work up.

Exercise

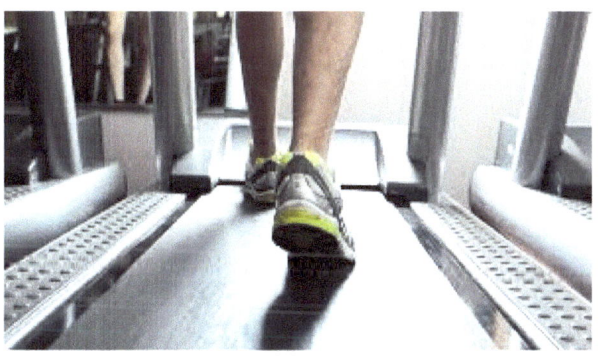

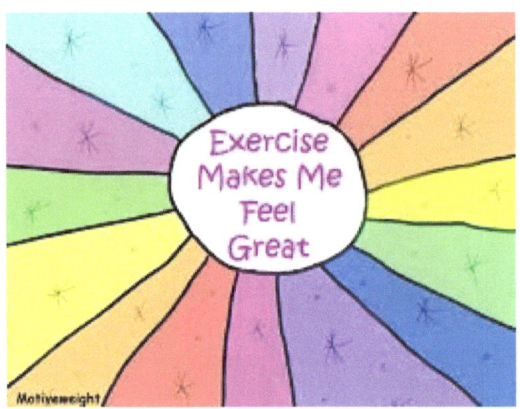

Pictures and facts courtesy of Shutter Stock on the web

www.ingramcontent.com/pod-product-compliance
Lightning Source LLC
Chambersburg PA
CBHW050432180526
45159CB00006B/2512